Don't Buy These Processed Foods!

This book is proudly presented
By
Lazaros Georgoulas
Independent Researcher and Author
lazageo@gmail.com

ISBN-13: 978-1499324372
ISBN-10: 1499324375

Copyright © Lazaros Georgoulas
Free to share, copy, modify, adapt!

Printed by CreateSpace, An Amazon.com company

"YOU ARE WHAT YOU EAT..."
A quote derived from many philosophies and religious systems from all around the world.

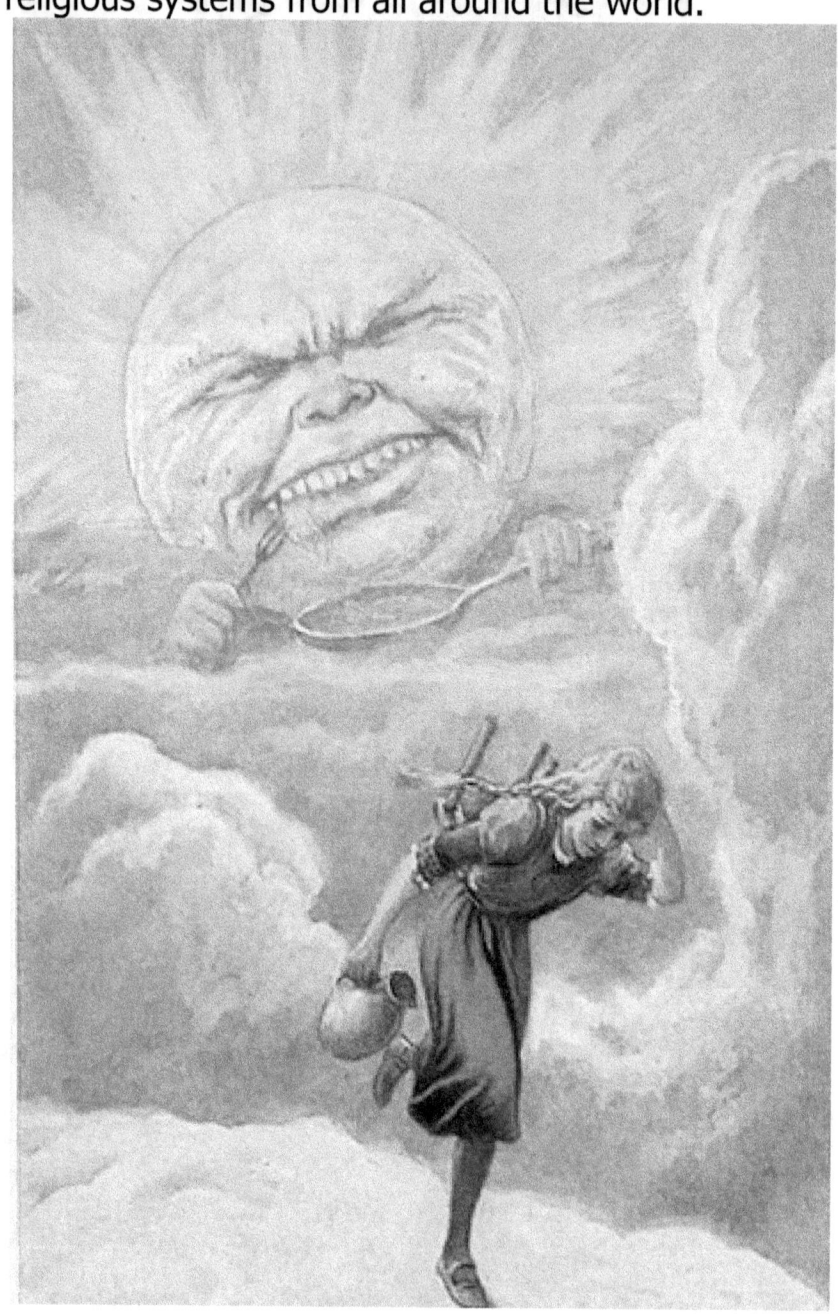

Have a look at this video revealing a secret way to lose weight (unlike anything you've seen before):

http://hyperdeals.biz/go/10/

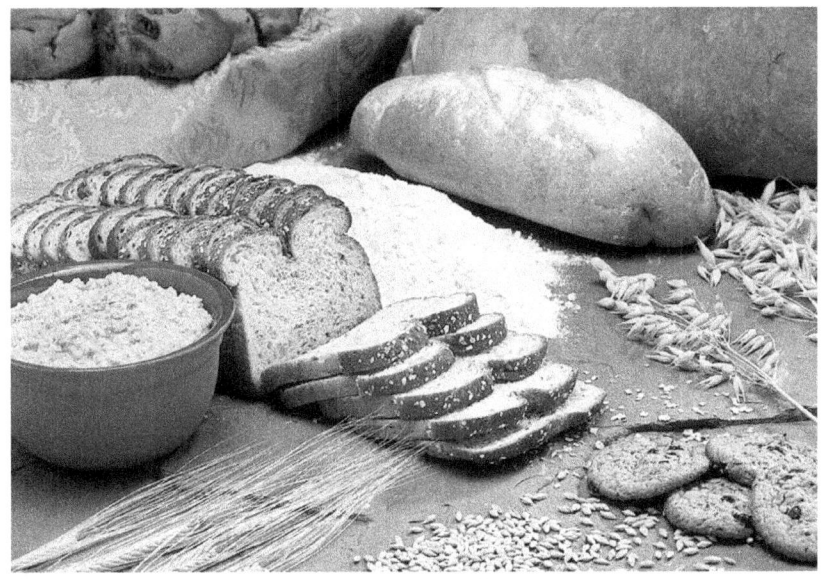

Table of Contents

Introduction

Bad Processed Food #1: French fries

Bad Processed Food #2: Chicken Nuggets

Bad Processed Food #3: Soda

Bad Processed Food #4: Processed Meats

Bad Processed Food #5: Fried Stuff in General

Bad Processed Food #6: Various types of Chips

Bad Processed Food #7: Cereals with Sugar

Bad Processed Food #8: Hamburgers and food from... Fast Foods!

Bad Processed Food #9: The well known Granola bars!

Bad Processed Food #10: Packed cookies, cakes, muffins, crackers etc.

Bad Processed Food #11: Deadly Margarine!

Bad Processed Food #12: Microwave food like Microwave Pop-corn!

Bad Processed Food #13: Flavored Tea!

Closing

Credits

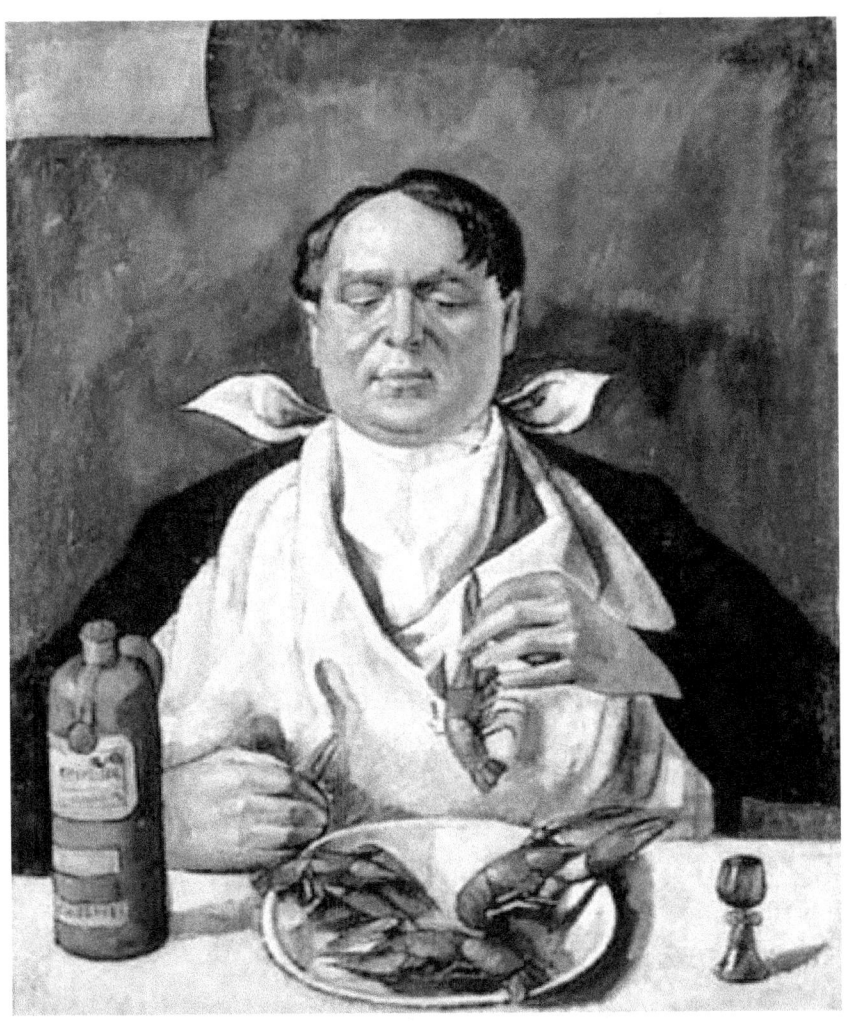

<u>Introduction</u>

Isn't food one of the most significant factors for the well-being of every human on Earth? Of course, this is a rhetoric question (one without the need for an answer!) and we all know (more or less) that food is important. It is said that for most people on Earth, food is the major subject for discussion every day.

"*You are what you eat...*" - How many times have you heard of this quote? I find it powerful and so true. If you eat junk then the whole body is filled with junk-ingredients (e.g. toxins). On the other hand if you eat healthy foods (e.g. 100% natural organic foods) your whole body will function better, you will feel rejuvenated and with a boosted self-confidence.

In this mini book I will present the worst processed foods for your health and the health of your loved ones, your family and/or friends. I recommend you avoid these processed foods like hell! I have investigated the issue by visiting certain processing food companies and here are the results of my investigation...

The worse processed foods ever (***DO NOT BUY THESE***)

These foods have the benefit of being tasty, sweet and they can be prepared in no time so they become the ideal meal for business people or people with not enough time for cooking. Some of the foods can become so addictive and the best we can do to help our body is avoid these foods! Because they might fill your stomach but they will harm your system in the long run...

Also, these particular foods are promoted by the media and this is why they are hard to resist eating them. They are usually low priced so people can buy them with no hesitation. But does strong health have a cost? Of course, not! So, even if you find it difficult to get rid of those specific processed foods from your diet, you got nothing to lose by trying.

But let's discover what these foods are...

Bad Processed Food #1: French fries

This is considered one of the most fattening foods out there (very high in calories). Scientists say that if you eat them regularly, you increase chances for diabetes to appear. Also, you put weight that it will be easy to lose. If you really like this food (most people do), eat the potato baked or even better read the following advice:

Important info: Personally, I am a fried potatoes lover, I really enjoy and desire this food. I know that many people enjoy it too. This is why I have researched the subject and written a mini book about how to turn normal unhealthy French fries into your healthiest food. You can find the book in my author's page on Amazon, click:
http://amazon.com/author/lazarosgeorgoulas/

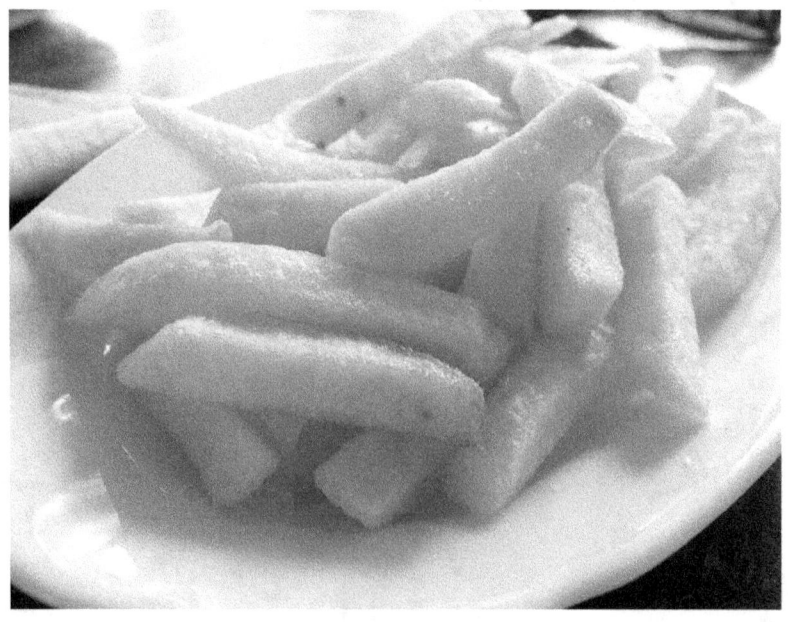

Bad Processed Food #2: Chicken Nuggets

Believe it or not this is one of the most desirable and tasty food these days (not only in USA but in every civilized place of our planet). They are very addictive and can easily satisfy a person's hunger in no time... BUT ...I went to the supermarket to search for some pre-made frozen chicken nuggets to cook and I was amazed by reading the ingredients on the product label... Too much salt, preservatives, fat and more worthless substances... Always look at the ingredients contained in the processed food you buy. Try to explore natural alternatives which are always present in supermarkets but not in the shelf in front of you. If you want to find them, you have to explore those supermarket shelves that are beyond or above the eye-level ;)

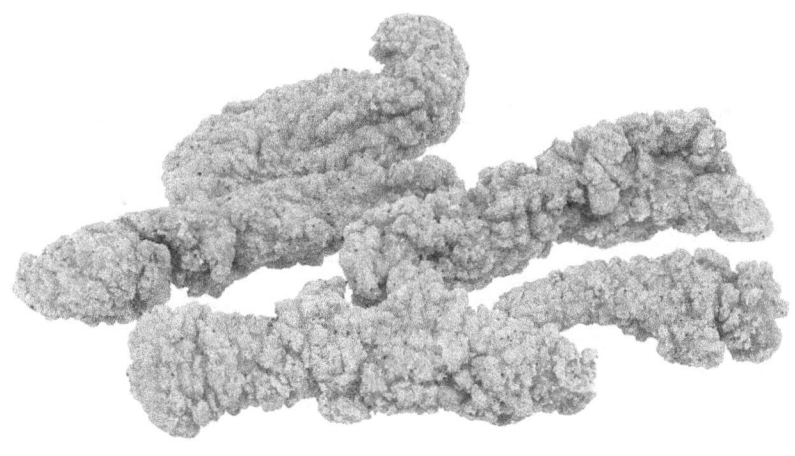

Bad Processed Food #3: Soda

With nothing but empty calories and with no nutritional value, Soda is one of the processed foods you should avoid!

I've also found that some types of Soda contain various syrups like corn fructose which beats plain sugar easily, in the race for the most unhealthy food of all!

Moreover there's a rumor that Soda is responsible for damaging Liver cells. It also affects blood pressure.

There's more. the Queen of Japan herself announced in the media that some foods are not to be consumed by people of the new era... Soda was among those foods. She also released an international press release mentioning the dangers from consuming certain processed foods or drinks. She said she did this for the good of humanity...

But no matter what the Queen of Japan says, if you want to do yourself a favor please avoid Soda!

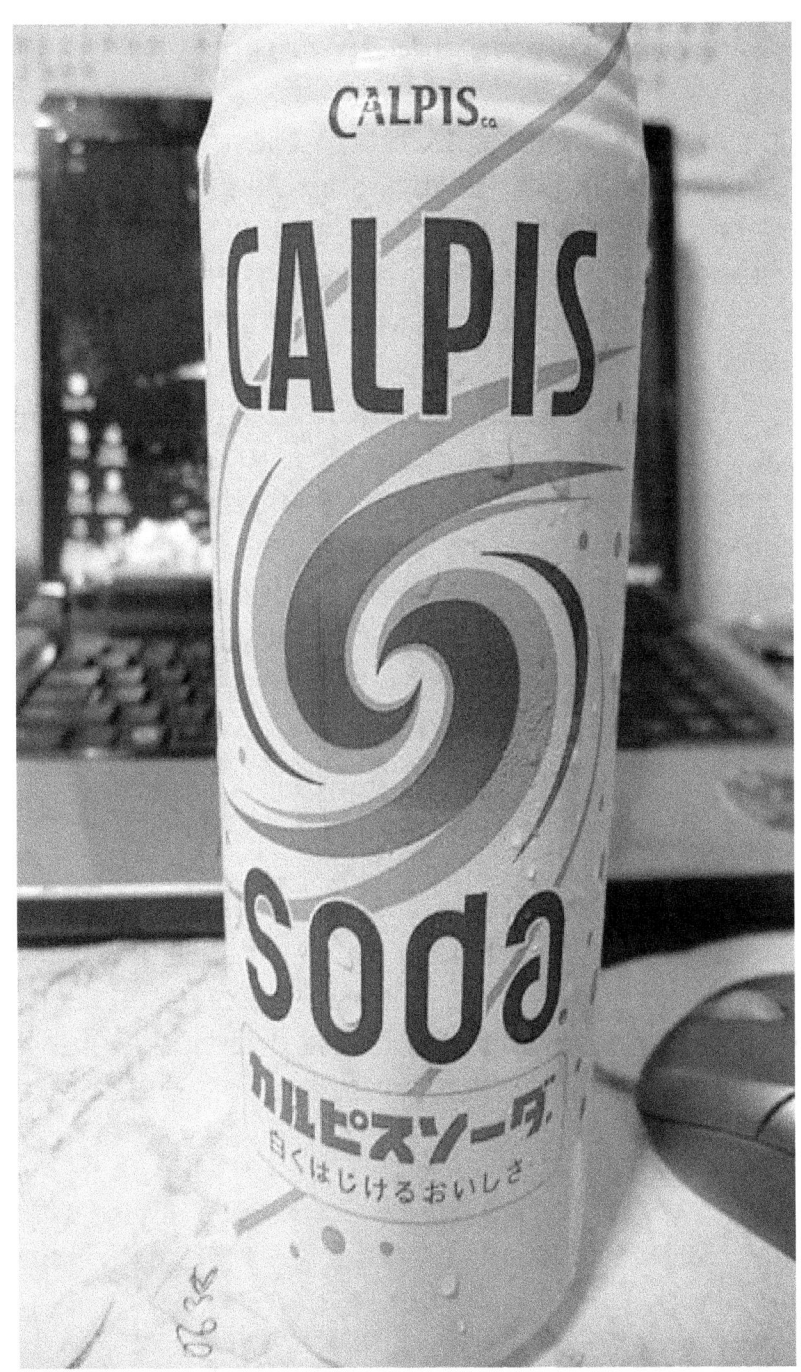

Bad Processed Food #4: Processed Meats

All processed meats you find in the market contain tons of artificial flavor ingredients, chemical preservatives, too much salt and other unwanted substances that I prefer not to mention here in order to prevent you from puking on this book!

The best advice when you want to buy processed meat is to read the ingredients in the back side of the product label. Food processing companies are required by law to write every single ingredient that was used in processing the meat. Including all those harmful substances and preservatives. They write these with really small fonts but they are readable.

You should consult the back side of every product label in detail so that you know what you eat! Especially when it comes to meat.

A friend who worked on a food processing factory told me once that the meat is processed under extreme pressure and in increased temperature. As a result the final meat product has lost much of its nutritional value...

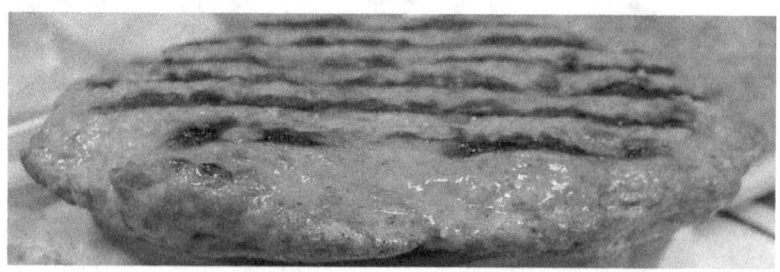

Bad Processed Food #5: Fried Stuff in General

If you are eating a lot of fried snacks then you should expect to gain weight easily. All those tasty snacks are so harmful in reality. A top food expert told me that most quick packed fried snacks out there (like potato chips) contain tons of empty calories, salt or sugar or both, preservatives and more. With no nutritional value at all, most fried stuff will ruin any efforts to lose weight and in no way they can promote a strong health. Moreover, these foods contain little or no fiber which means they can be difficult to digest. An advice would be to eat those bad foods along with other foods that contain fibers (e.g. some fresh bread or 100% pure cereals)

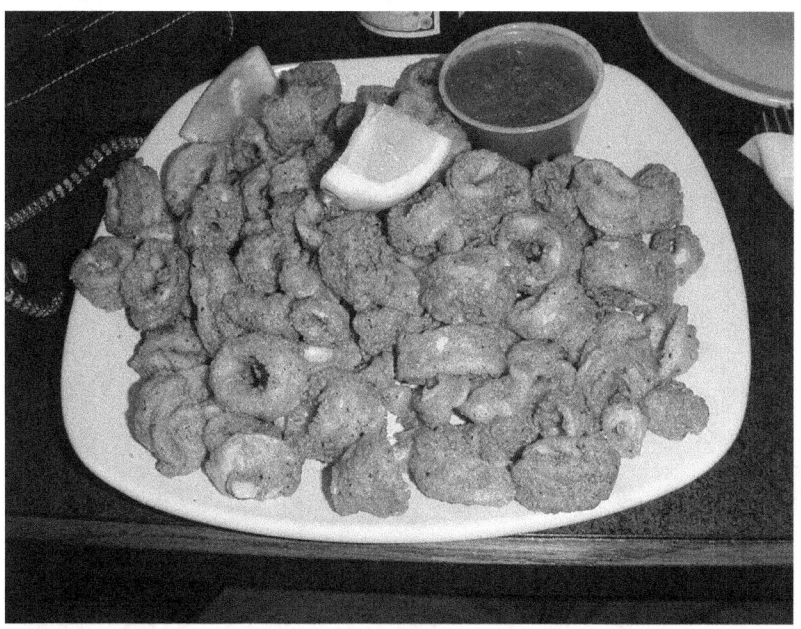

Bad Processed Food #6: Various types of Chips

I know I referred to French Fries and fried foods in general but there are so many types of Chips out there that your really want to avoid. Apart from the empty calories and the "Zero" nutritional value, these addictive salty devils are so d@mn fattening plus they contain all sorts of substances with really weird names. Look at the product label so that you know what you put in your stomach! Are you on a diet? Forget chips, they will ruin it. Do you want to maintain strong health so as to conquer all your goals in life? YES! If you are not strong as a rock how else you will achieve your highest dreams and desires in life? So, no more chips please or at least eat them only in rare occasions. Stop torturing yourself.

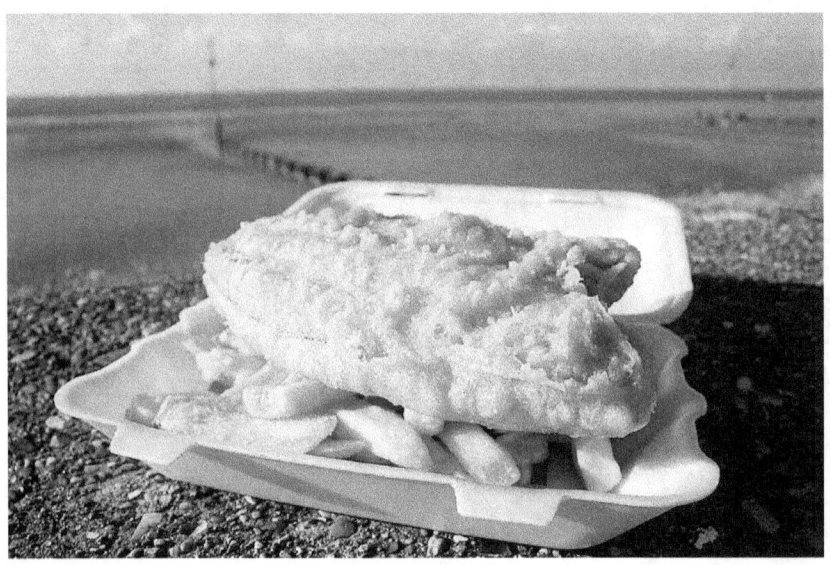

Bad Processed Food #7: Cereals with Sugar

Another food that represents a leading cause of obesity and its harmful effects. What's even more frightening is that we eat those cereals in the morning just before we start the survival for the day.

How ironic?

Instead of eating something that will boost our health and performance we eat those sweet cereals. They are fattening (looooots of sugar) and lead to the severe health situation of Diabetes if consumed regularly.

If you enjoy eating cereals because you know they are rich in fibers then choose 100% naturally processed cereals with no sugar or other additives.

I know, I know it's hard to find those but it's worth the trouble. Your health has no price!

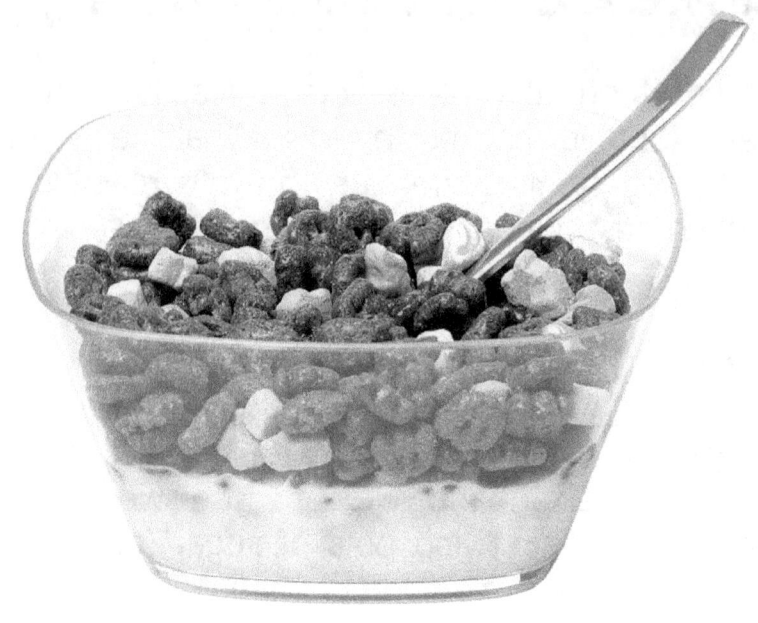

Have a look at this video (if still active) revealing a secret way to lose weight (unlike anything you've seen before):

http://hyperdeals.biz/go/10/

Bad Processed Food #8: Hamburgers and food from... Fast Foods!

You knew I was going to say something about those hamburgers you enjoy so much right? Yes indeed they are tasty and so addictive but would you like to know how they are made and what additives they contain? Did you know most hamburgers contain blood from the animal as well as trimmed bones from the animal to enhance flavor (if you ask a food expert he/she will tell you that the best part of the meat, the one with the most flavor is the meat near the bone. Food companies (and I know this from an insider) do not throw away the bones or the blood from the slaughtered animals (excuse me for this tone of writing) BUT they use them along with lots of salt and other additives to create our wonderful and tasty hamburgers that we all desire every now and then...

So think twice before ordering a hamburger next time you go to the restaurant or fast food shop.

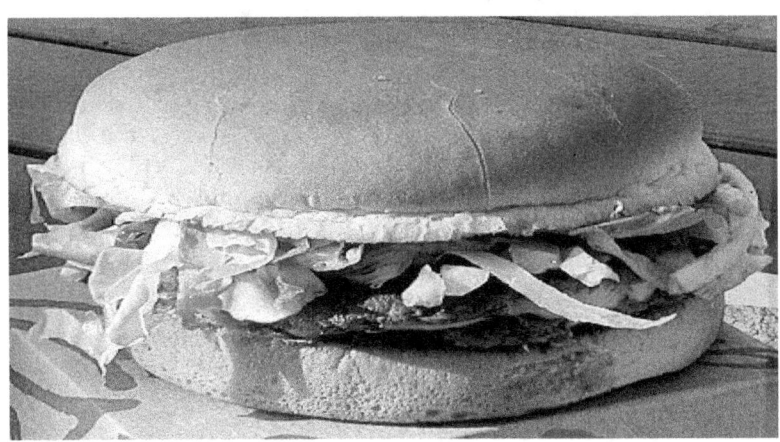

Bad Processed Food #9: The well known Granola bars!

Yeap, those nicely packed and so tasty snacks. Avoid them! Many of you might don't know this food although it is marketed like crazy in many countries. Consider it like any bar like a chocolate bar or honey bar etc. All those bars contain excessive fats, sugar, HFCS to enhance sweetness and more (you don't want to know). To realize in what extend do preservatives are added in those bars have a closer look at the ingredients (usually listed with tiny letters but still readable). I wonder, why do they have to add so many weird ingredients in a plain chocolate or Granola bar... Anyway, avoid these bars and you will have a better immune system to avoid health situations like diabetes.

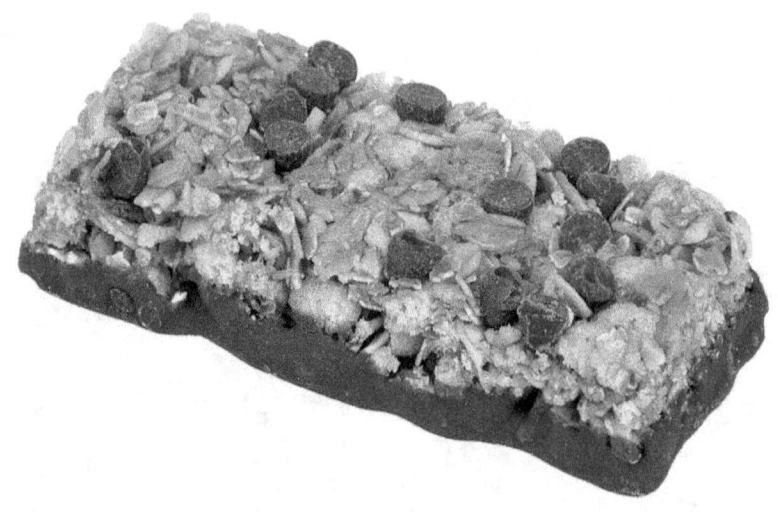

Bad Processed Food #10: Packed cookies, cakes, muffins, crackers etc.

I know, I know we are talking about really desirable foods here. I enjoy eating those lovely cookies every now and then but wait until you find out what these foods contain. High level of sugar and/or salt of unknown quality (usually deeply processed sugar and salt). A great effort has been made by food companies producing these goodies to "Hide" the harmful effects with a nice well marketed appearance. You will usually find these lethal foods in beautiful packages (e.g. TV commercial). These foods have really nice shapes making them so adorable. I know. I only want you to do one thing. Read all the ingredients the packed food contains. Aim for the more natural ones. Avoid chemical substances added to prolong the expiry date of the food. Avoid the marketing. Trust your instinct especially when it comes to eating such food...

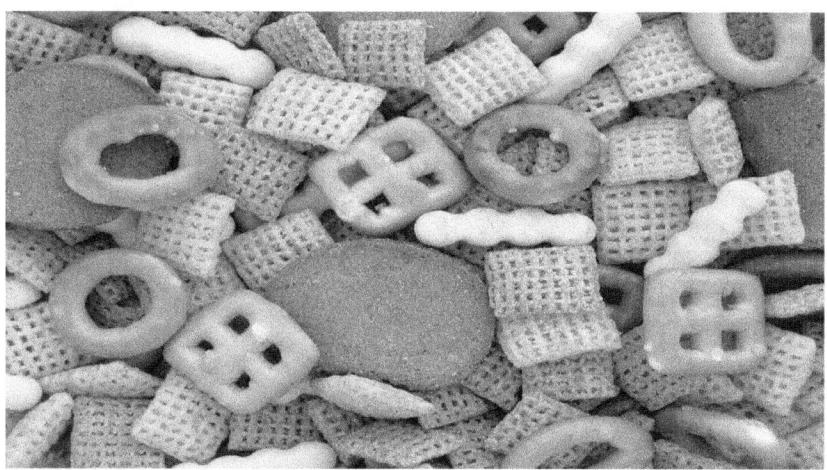

Bad Processed Food #11: Deadly Margarine!

Margarine is a very popular alternative for butter. A lot of people consume it especially in morning hours. Margarine contains lots of fats, salt, preservatives, emulsifiers, *Hexane* possibly. Just read the ingredients and you will be amazed. Funny thing is that Margarine is promoted as a healthy food. As a food that will keep us "alive and kicking" throughout the day. What a myth! Do not consume margarine regularly unless you want to be faced with serious health issues like cancer, diabetes or obesity. Do not believe the false claims that Margarine is THE most appropriate food to begin your day with. When in the super-market do not be tempted to buy it remembering those shiny Margarine TV ads you saw the other day. Look behind the scenes... How? Read all the ingredients contained in the food. Why not make this a habit for every processed food you buy?

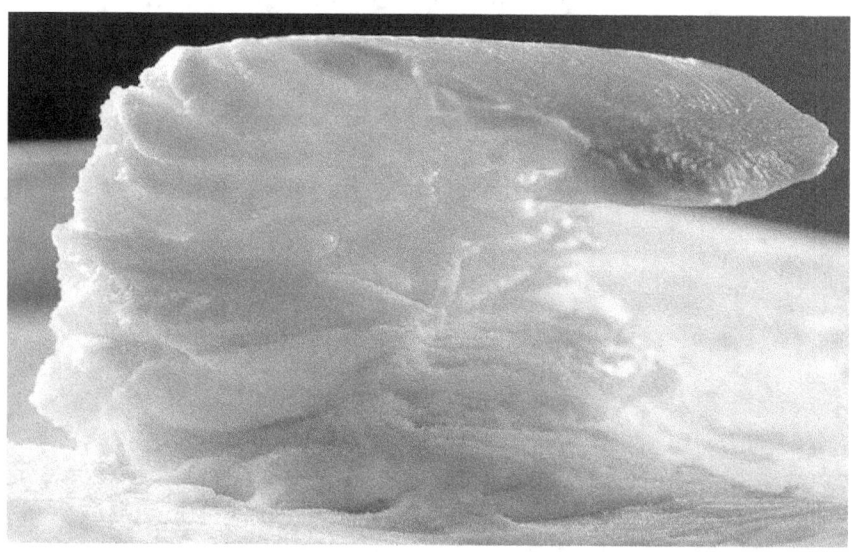

Bad Processed Food #12: Microwave food like Microwave Pop-corn!

Here we are talking about one of the most popular and most marketed foods in the industry.

Microwave pop-corn!

We've all tried it in the cinema or at home while watching our favorite show on TV.

First thing you need to know about this food is that it is produced from low quality seeds that are genetically modified (Man's madness to become God).

Second, it is packed with lots of salt and weird chemicals and preservatives to prolong expiry date. One such chemical is *Diatecyl* which is known to cause damage to lungs.

If you want to eat pop-corn it would be really wise to prepare it yourself.

It is so easy and you can make it 100 times more healthy than any industrial pop-corn. So make it a habit to cook your own pop-corn.

Same applies for every pre-made meal that only needs heating with microwaves (they will destroy it even more). Stay away from these foods as much as you can.

Science will soon declare microwaves as harmful for the quality of the food and for the humans who consume it!

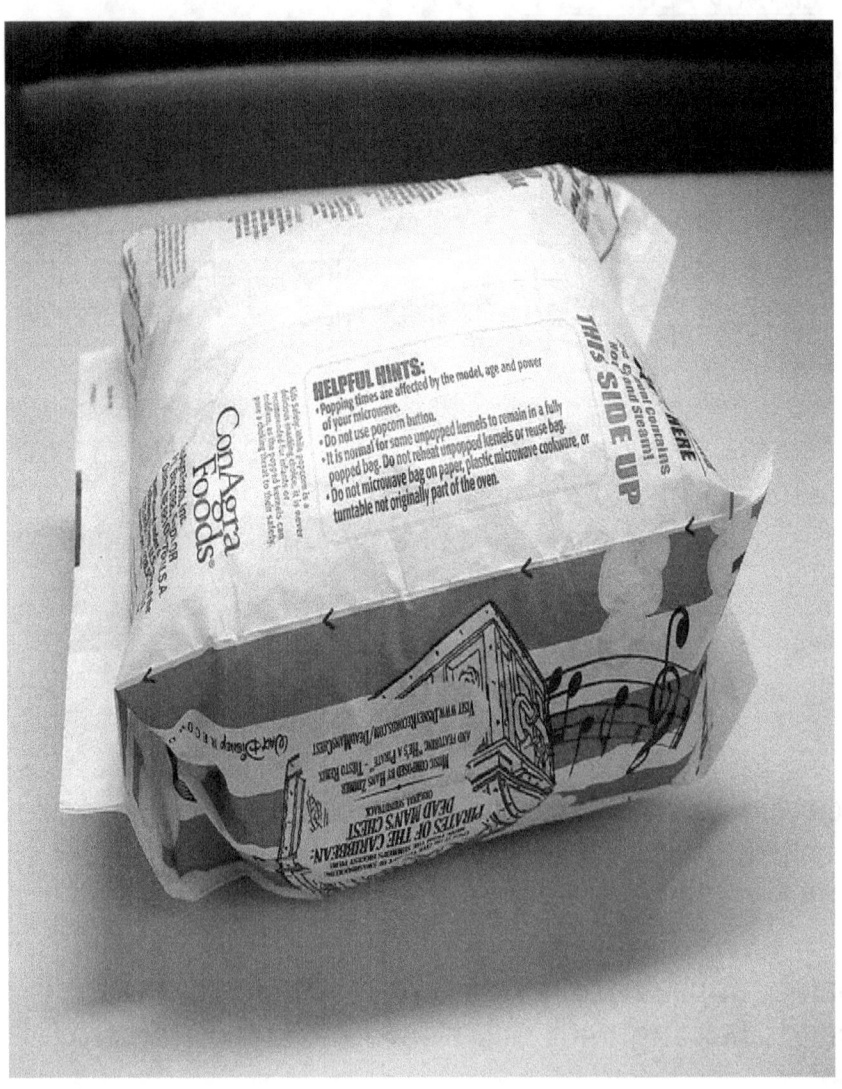

Bad Processed Food #13: Flavored Tea!

I kept this for last because it is so addictive and funny thing is that many athletes consume it. But it can be a lot more harmful than you can imagine. I am talking about processed Tea drinks like iced Tea or Tea mixes. These are usually marketed very well and they are quite cheap so anyone can buy them and become addicted to them! But do know that most flavor is artificial no matter what they tell you in the TV commercial... These drinks are totally empty with no nutritional value at all. They increase thirst instead of resolving it because they contain various sugars. Read the label with the ingredients. Check out the percentage of real/genuine tea that is contained in the drink. It should be under 1%!

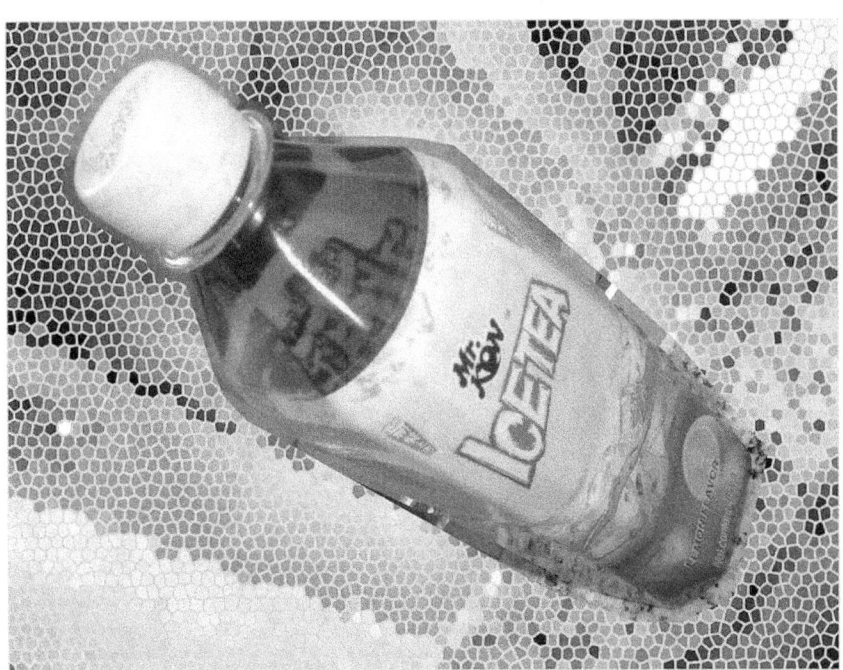

And that's the worst processed foods you should never buy.-

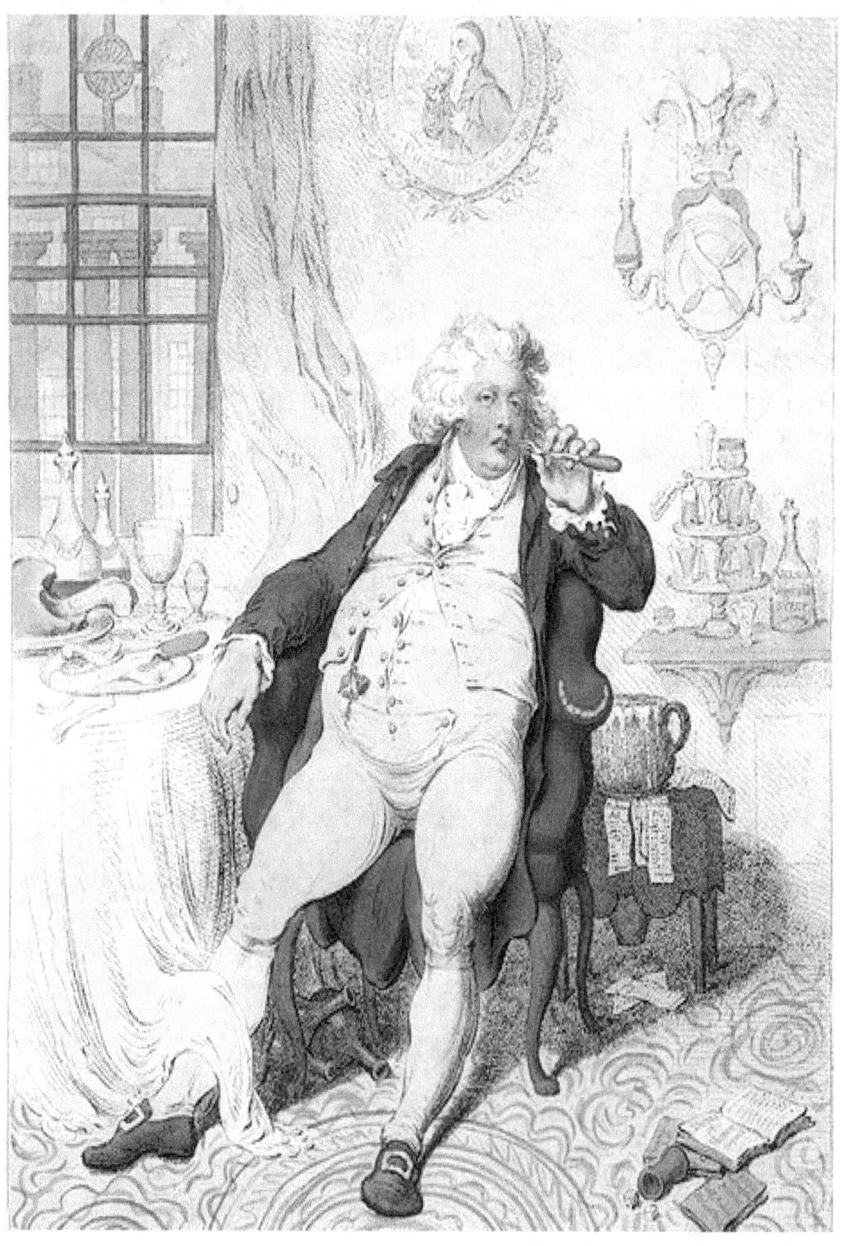

__Closing__...

If you want to be strong as a rock you want to maintain a great health. By avoiding or measuring the consumption of the foods I mentioned in this book, you will increase your overall health and well being. You will be more productive and you will start to develop a healthier lifestyle. I hope I gave you some insights through this book.

Before I leave you I want to share one more detail with you. You should also avoid all kinds of fat free foods... In general the less a food is processed the better it's quality. But when it comes to fat-free or sugar-free foods or drinks just keep in mind that there's a lot of processing going on and a lot of unwanted substances included in the whole mixture to produce the drink that gives us so much temporal excitement but in the long run it can become really harmful and lead to severe health situations. So, what is the secret key?

You know what ancient Greeks used to say? "*Consume everything you like, either good or bad, either in the physical or the spiritual world but always know your limits...*"

This quote tells us that it is hard to resist some of the foods mentioned in this mini book. But if you are about to eat them at least don't cross the line.

Do not eat them often or eat them in small portions. You will do yourself a great favor and you will stay alive and kicking for many years to come!

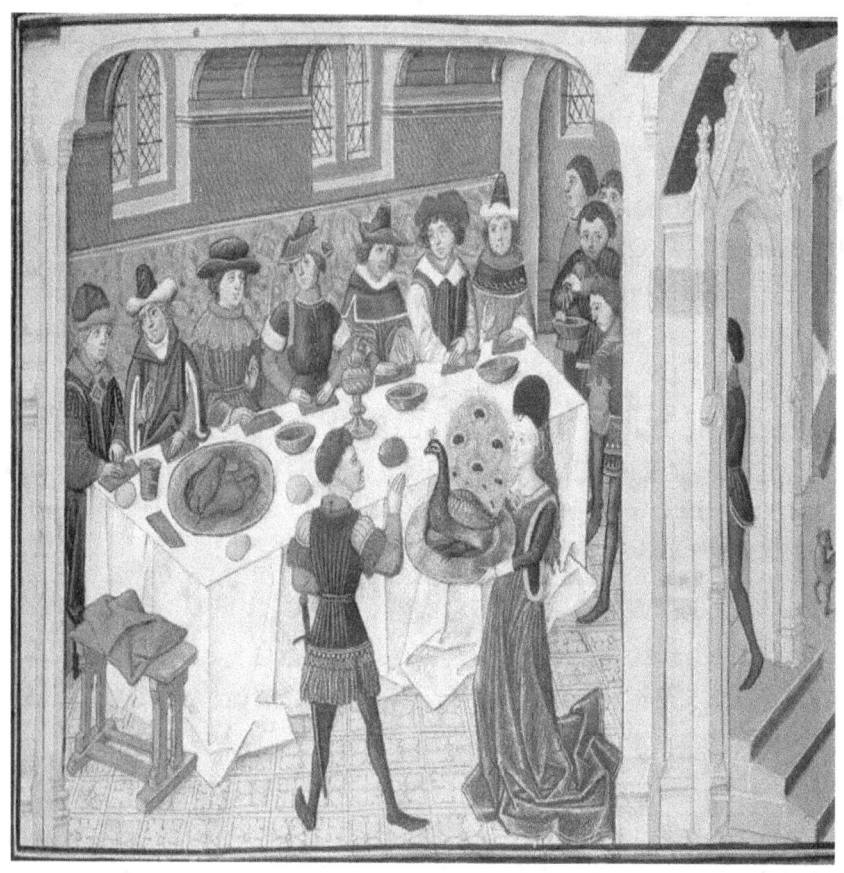

I hope you enjoyed this mini book. If so, please leave an honest review on Amazon. Here's my author page I also have other books (kindle and paperback) there:

http://amazon.com/author/lazarosgeorgoulas/

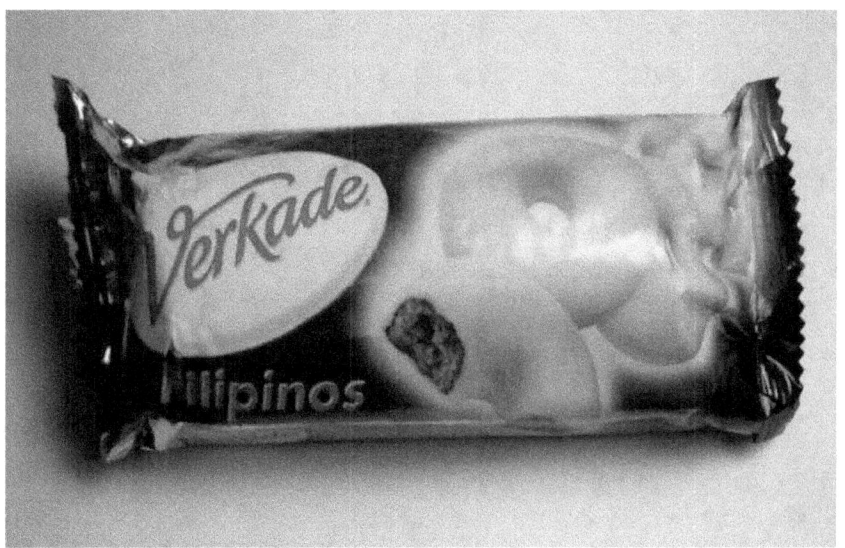

Credits

First I want to thank my editor and close friend Maria Markella. I love you Maria. Check her author profile in Amazon, she has some interesting books there:

http://amazon.com/author/mariamarkella/

This book is distributed and protected under this Creative Commons License:
http://creativecommons.org/licenses/by-sa/3.0/

All images from Wikimedia Commons:
http://commons.wikimedia.com

Biso - http://commons.wikimedia.org/wiki/File:Chipsqw.JPG
Evan-Amos - http://commons.wikimedia.org/wiki/File:McD-Chicken-Selects.jpg
http://commons.wikimedia.org/wiki/File:Chewy-Granola-Bar.jpg
Cliff Cheng LF - http://commons.wikimedia.org/wiki/File:Calpis_Soda.jpg
http://commons.wikimedia.org/wiki/File:A_fried_calamari.jpg
Andrew Dunn - http://commons.wikimedia.org/wiki/File:Fish_and_chips.jpg
Ericd - http://commons.wikimedia.org/wiki/File:Hamburger_sandwich.jpg
Helge Höpfner - http://commons.wikimedia.org/wiki/File:FD_2.jpg
Howcheng - http://commons.wikimedia.org/wiki/File:Popcorn_bag_popped.jpg
MasterHonCFoo2 - http://commons.wikimedia.org/wiki/File:MasterKongCom_MrKonIceTea2.jpg
Oskar Herrfurth - http://www.goethezeitportal.de/wissen/illustrationen/legenden-maerchen-und-sagenmotive/das-maerchen-von-den-sieben-raben-herrfurth.html
http://commons.wikimedia.org/wiki/File:Verkade_Filipinos_Wit_1.jpg

YOUR NOTES...:

Would you like more from Lazaros **Georgoulas**? See his author page on Amazon, click:
http://amazon.com/author/lazarosgeorgoulas/

Here's the author page of my lovely editor **Maria Markella:**
http://amazon.com/author/mariamarkella/

Some great offers (if still valid):

Have a look at this video revealing a secret way to lose weight (unlike anything you've seen before): http://hyperdeals.biz/go/10/

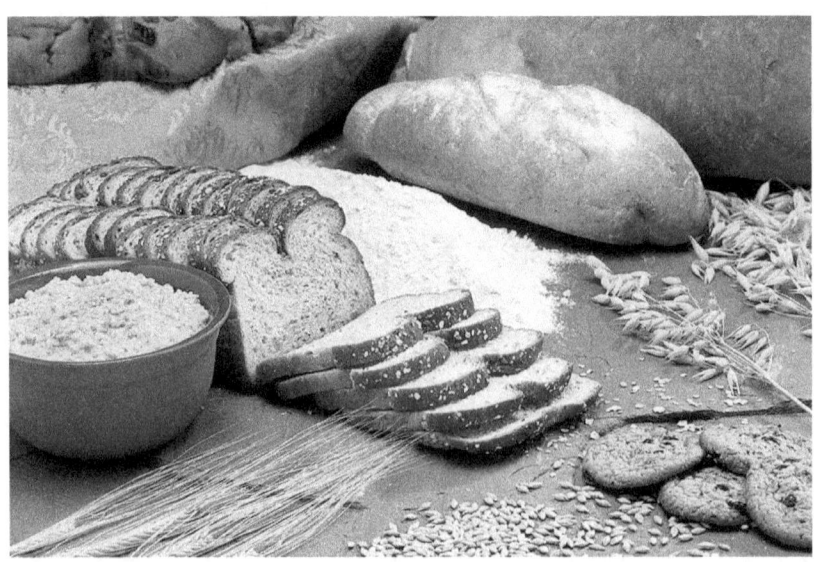

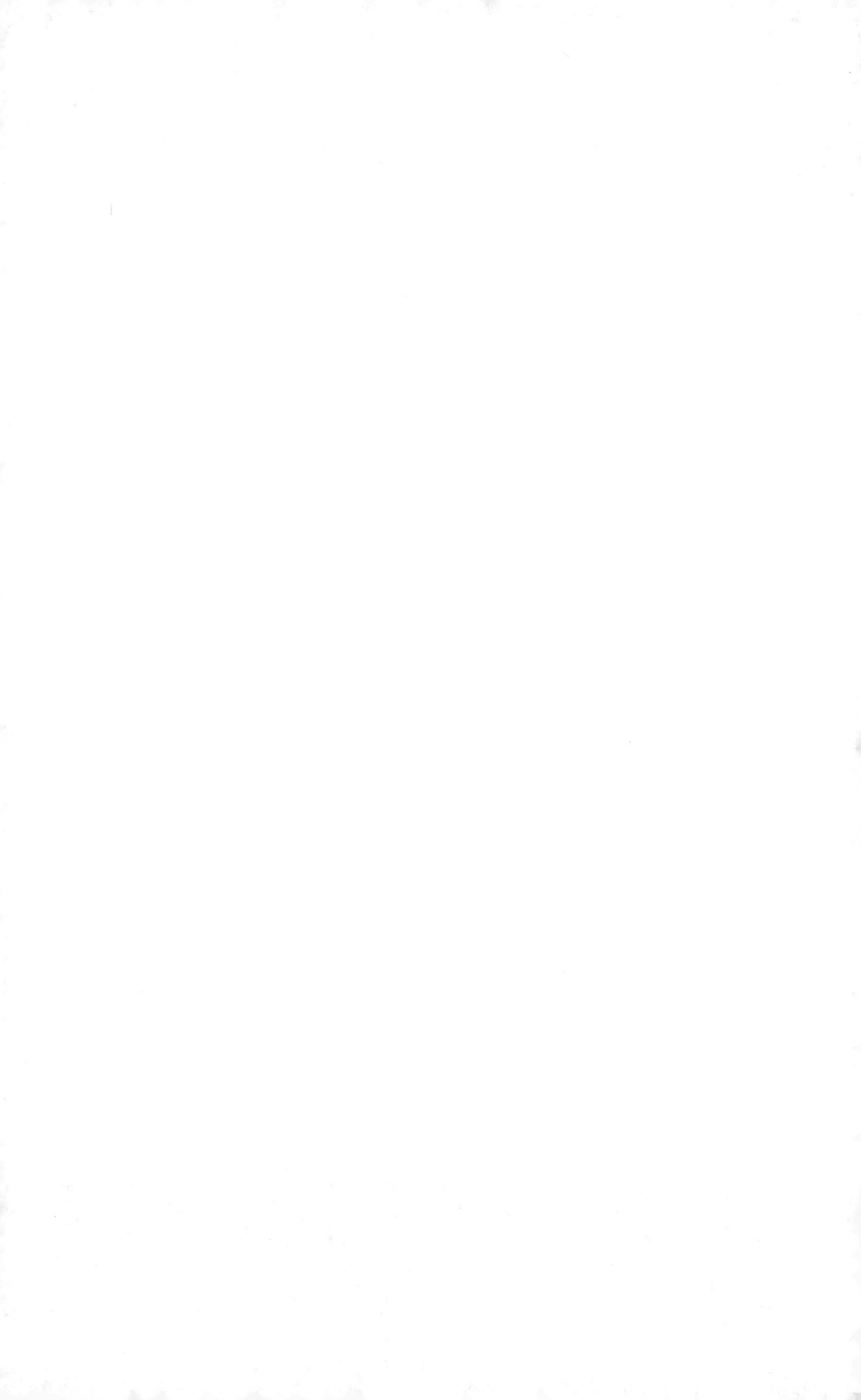

www.ingramcontent.com/pod-product-compliance
Lightning Source LLC
Chambersburg PA
CBHW060445290526
45793CB00002B/578